Sex Guide

50 High Definition Sex Positions That Guarantees A Scream From Your Woman

MATT ELTON

Limit of Liability

The information in this book is solely for informational
purposes, not as a medical instruction to replace the advice of
your physician or as a replacement for any treatment prescribed
by your physician. The author and publisher do not take
responsibility for any possible consequences from any treatment,
procedure, exercise, dietary modification, action or application of
medication which results from reading or following the
information contained in this book.

If you are ill or suspect that you have a medical problem, we
strongly encourage you to consult your medical, health, or other
competent professional before adopting any of the suggestions
in this book or drawing inferences from it.

This book and the author's opinions are solely for informational
and educational purposes. The author specifically disclaims all
responsibility for any liability, loss, or risk, personal or otherwise
which is incurred as a consequence, directly or indirectly, of the
use and application of any of the contents of this book.

ISBN-13: 978-1530033980

ISBN-10: 1530033985

DEDICATION

To all who desire to live life to the fullest!

TABLE OF CONTENT

INTRODUCTION

Now this book was made just for you. Buying this book is one great and revolutionary step towards a great sex life, now don't mind me; I know you may have bought other good stuffs too. This is one book that is founded by a great passion to see couples enjoy new and creative sex the way I do.

Many couples just oscillate between the regular missionary position and maybe one or two more sex positions and it's becoming something to worry about as they are getting tired of regular stuffs, and it is really becoming boring to them. They are getting tired of how limited those few sex positions can be.

You made a great choice downloading this book. Enjoy as you read through its pages and have fun as much as I did when I was putting up the bits and pieces of this book up. Have great fun with your partners. Have fun as you read.

Butterfly Sex Position

The sex position is an advanced sexual position in which the woman lies on a low table, ottoman, or a bed and lifts her legs onto her partner's shoulders. The now supports her hips to allow for proper positioning.

The butterfly sex position is a really great position to do if the couples are looking for a way to liven up their sex life or they just want to try sex in a different location or room. They should ensure that the object they use is stable, and sturdy, and can handle some rough play. Enjoy.

Reverse cowgirl

The man lies on his back and, while facing his feet the woman straddles him with her knees on either side of his hips. Or, if it's more comfortable, she should squat over him with her feet flat on the bed. When he's nice and hard (and of course when the woman's vagina is well lubricated), the woman places one hand on the bed or on his legs to steady herself, as she holds the base of his penis with her other hand, and slowly lower herself onto him.

Once he's securely inside of her, she starts moving up and down, using her leg muscles to build momentum. The woman can help maintain her balance by placing her hands in front of her (on his legs or the bed), or reach back and put her hands on his thighs. One of the major advantages of any girl-on-top position: the woman is in control, so she mixes things up and does whatever she feels best. She can vary the speed and depth of penetration. Or play with her movements by gyrating back and forth or in circles instead of just up and down. At some point, the woman should try arching her back, which allows his member to stimulate her G-spot. And, since the woman has easy access to her clitoris, she should give herself a hand if you need it.

Lap Dance Sex Position

This position has a lot of resemblance to the Back Seat Driver Sex position. This is a sex position where the man can really relax and 'enjoy the show' the same way he would almost not do anything in a strip club, though he has the option of being more active.

The man sits on a comfortable seat or sofa. He should sit far back in the sofa or seat and should also have his legs open wide. The woman will be on her feet and need to back up into her man. She needs to get a hold of his penis and guide it in to her vagina. Once he is in safely, she can choose to either grind slowly on her man while he stays deep inside of her OR she can choose to bounce up and bounce down on top of him with his penis deep inside OR the man can help his woman using his arms OR she can choose to lean forwards or backwards on her man, depending on how intimate the couple intends to make the lap dance sex position.

Deep Impact Sex Position

This sex position is a variation of the Deep Stick sex position, but it is easier as the man kneels by the side of the bed or couch thereby lining up more easily with the woman. To get into position, the woman lies on her back with her legs resting on the shoulders of the man, who penetrates his woman from a kneeling position. This position also stays true to its name, meaning the man can thrust in with all intensity, unless of course he is too big. Any height difference or discomforts on the side of the man can be easily be fixed using pillows.

Downstroke Sex Positions

This position is also a variation of the Deep Stick sex position, but it is easier as the man crouches by the side of the bed, sofa or couch. So he lines up more easily with the woman. To get into this position, the woman will need to lie on her back with her legs resting on the shoulders of the man, the man then penetrates from a standing position. But due to the higher position of the man this variation is not as intimate as either the Deep Stick sex position or its other family the Deep Impact sex position.

Jockey Sex Position

This position got its name from the idea that your man would like a horse riding jockey when in this position.

The woman lies with her face downwards on her bed with her legs together and straight. The man now straddles her with his knees on either side of her waist. The man then enters the woman either anally or vaginally and starts to thrust. He doesn't have to lean forward as a jockey would do when riding a race horse but he can if he wanted. He can also lean backwards slightly in the Jockey position. The man can also lean right on top of her so that it feels more like you are spooning with him.

Drill Sex Position

In this position, the woman lies on her back and wraps her legs around her man who mounts her from above. Although it looks very similar to the Missionary position, the raised legs of the woman makes a significant improvement in the penetration angle as well as the intimacy, therefore making it a good first step for improving the sometimes monotonous starting position.

Exposed Eagle Sex Position

This position might just be one of the hardest positions to perform. It requires great flexibility and strength. If you don't have this gym or yoga expertise, then the couple is in for a pretty sore time!

The best way to get into this position is to start out in the Cowgirl position. This means that the woman needs to be on top of her man with her knees on either side of him. She then lies backwards until her back is resting on her man's thighs and knees while she is still on her knees. He can raise his knees if she isn't flexible enough so she is more upright. The man now needs to raise his upper body so that he is in a seated position. He can then put his arms behind him to support himself or he can put them around the woman's back.

Hang Loose Sex Position

This position is really an easy one to perform. It is a variation of the regular Missionary position. You don't have to sleep in the gym or be a work out expert to get into this position

The couple starts off in the regular Missionary position, instead of them lying with their heads by where the pillows are and their feet near the end of the bed, the couple lies across the bed. Lying across the bed will give both of them far less space. To overcome this, the woman should position herself so that her head and part of her shoulders are hanging over the edge of the bed. Her man will also be hanging over the bed, so he will need to extend his arms outwards and put his hands on the ground to support himself.

This sex position got its name from the fact that the couples are literally hanging over the edge of your bed.

Italian Hanger Sex Position

This sex position is great for hitting the woman's G-Spot while, and she also has a cool 'exposed' and slightly submissive feeling to it. It is very easy to make a transition from the missionary position into the Italian Hanger. The woman just needs to lie on her back

As the man is having the regular missionary sex, he would then need to get to his knees and bring them quite close to the woman, which will force her legs apart. When he is on his knees, he then needs to put his hands under the woman's bum and hips and lift them up. To help him out with raising her bum and hips, the woman bends her knees and plant her feet on the bed. This will allow her to push her waist or hips into the air.

The launch Pad sex position

It is one great way to get into a synchronistic sexual flow, whether the couple opts for deep and powerful thrusts or gentle rocking. It's also helps if couples want to achieve deep penetration and the massage of the woman's G-spot.

As in Deep Stick sex position, the woman lies on her back and raises her hips; the man now kneels down in front. Once the man penetrates the woman and begins to thrust, the woman's hips rise and fall in beautiful rhythm to every thrust. A positional aid can be placed underneath the buttocks of the woman, to help her maintain the elevation of her hips.

The woman's leg positions can be modified in many ways, like: bringing both legs over to a side, the man raising them over his shoulders, or keeping her feet together and spreading her knees wide. The woman can also place her feet on the chest of her man to bear some of his weight so that her man can lean over top of her legs; this gives a difference in sensation.

Missionary 180 Sex Position

This Sex Position is like a combination of two sex positions, the regular Missionary and the Betty Rocker Sex positions. For the man it will require quite a bit of flexibility in his penis to be able perform the position.

11

The woman starts by lying down on her back with her legs fairly spread out. The man will then lie down on top of her. But instead of the couples lying facing each other, the man will be lying head-to-toe with his legs spread out, resting on either side of you on the bed. The man now slowly and carefully pushes his penis downwards so that he can thrust into the woman's vagina. This will definitely put a lot of strain on the suspensory ligaments in the man's penis, hence the need for a reasonable level of flexibility, so he needs to be extra careful while doing this.

Pirate's Bounty Sex Position

In this sex position, the woman lies on her back with one of her legs resting on the man's shoulder; the other leg is wrapped around the man's thigh (the ship mast). The man penetrates her vagina from a kneeling position. Fairly easier to perform than its near cousin the Deep Stick, this position holds true to its name, meaning that the man can penetrate with every ounce of strength he has, unless of course he is too big. Any genital altitude difference should be corrected easily, by the use of pillows.

The Playing Of the Cello Sex Position

This position is a really enjoyable one for the woman. The reason it has the name is because the man will look almost like he is playing the cello with the woman's legs.

The woman lies on her back and raises her legs so that the legs are pointing towards the ceiling. Her man is then positioned upright, on his knees and penetrates the woman while facing her. The woman now rests both of her legs on just one of his shoulders, either the right or the left shoulder. The man now wraps one arm around the woman's feet and lower leg, while wrapping his other arm around her thighs, which makes the man look like he's playing the cello with his woman's legs, hence the name playing the Cello sex position.

Right Angle Sex Position

It is a really easy to perform sex position and doesn't require so much flexibility.

The woman starts by lying down on her back and pointing her feet towards the ceiling. She doesn't have to worry so much about keeping her legs perfectly straight. The man then sits down on the bed with his legs spread open. He should be facing his woman and sitting down on the bed just below her vagina with his legs in front of him on either side of the woman's body. The man now grabs her legs and lifts her up and towards him. He can then thrust into her.

The Right Angle got its name from the idea that the couple will be making a 90 degree angle, which is a right angle with your bodies in this sex position.

Sandwich Sex Position

This position is a little like the combination if two sex positions, the Viennese Oyster and Drill positions. It requires a little bit of flexibility and strength on the part of the woman.

The woman lies down on her back and let her man thrust into her as he would while in the Missionary position; on top. But instead of just resting her legs on the bed like she would in the missionary, she brings them towards herself while keeping them open. Her man's arms should usually be around her shoulders on the bed, but he would now have to lower them so that he can put one under each of her knees and help her to lift them upwards to change the angle that he's thrusting her from.

Tug of Love Sex Position

This position is one of a kind, and the last thing couples might actually dream of.

The man first need to lie down on the bed on his back with his legs open. The woman then sits down on top of him and let him thrust into her vagina, with her legs on either side of him in front of her. Next She needs to start to lean backwards until she is lying down on the bed (she should put her arms behind her to ease herself down). Her head should be close to his feet. The woman can rest her legs on his chest or on either side of him, whichever is more comfortable.

Now that they are both lying down, the man should grab her hands so that he can pull her in towards him.

Victory Sex Position

The Victory is more or less the Missionary position but with the woman's legs extended out straight and forming into a v-shape toward the ceiling.

In this position, the woman simply lays down on her back while her partner lies face-down on top of her.

Viennese Oyster Sex Position

This sex position requires a great deal of flexibility. And most couples usually would get to a point where they can't continue due to the woman's inability to push past that point.

In this sex position the woman lays on her back with her lower back and legs raised all the way up so that her ankles are crossed behind her own head. The exact end position depends on the flexibility of the woman. This position totally exposes the groin of the woman to the man who lays on top the woman to penetrate. The man moves up and down on the woman to create friction. He needs to use his hands to support his own body weight so as not to crush his woman.

X Marks the Spot Sex Position

This sex position is really just a variation of the regular Missionary position. It's fun to try if the couple finds out that they are getting bored of Missionary and want something similar but more fun and different.

To perform it, the woman lays on her back while her man is on top. This position got its 'X' part from the fact that the bodies of the couples will form an X when viewed from above. So if the woman is lying down on her back with her feet at the end of the bed and her head at the top of the bed where the pillows usually are, her man will be lying across the bed, with his head by one side of the bed and his feet by the other side of the bed.

Bumper Cars Sex Position

This position is one very exotic position. To some couples this position is simple novel and to some others it is cool. Even the name is a little out of there.

The man must be sure to check that his penis is flexible enough. If he is standing up straight, then the man needs to be able to point his penis directly downwards towards the ground quite comfortably before even trying out this sex position.

If the man has enough flexibility, then you are good to go. Firstly the woman lies down on her stomach on the bed, with her legs straight and open wide. Then her man lies down on his stomach facing in completely the opposite direction and his legs straight and open wide as well. The man then reverses back towards the woman until his thighs are positioned over her thighs and he can pull his penis so that it's pointing towards her vagina. Then the man slowly needs penetrates the woman's vagina, making sure not to overstretch his penis.

Irish Garden Sex Position

The position is similar to the Betty Rocker position, very interesting and doesn't take a great deal of flexibility as it might look. It's very easy to perform.

The man sits down on the bed. He should have his back upright and straight, his legs out in front of him and also opened fairly wide. The man can bend his knees if he finds that more comfortable for him. The woman now gets down on all fours and reverses herself towards him. She will have to lower her waist down onto her man by straightening out her legs behind him (one on each side of his waist). Next she lowers her head and shoulders onto the bed until they are resting on it.

Doggie Style

This position also known as rear entry is a great position that has enjoyed popularity over the years, maybe because it comes with this naughty feeling.

In this position, the man enters the woman's vagina from behind as she is on all fours on the bed or couch. This position supports very deep penetration, as the woman's body is already being so angled; so the g-spot can be stimulated by each penetration of the man's penis. Depending on how far bent over the woman is and how fast the man can thrust into his woman. His testicles will also slap against his woman's vagina which can be really very exciting. Stimulation of the Clitoris is also very possible by both the partners.

Superwoman Sex Position

This position may sound like one of those positions where the woman literally needs to do alot of work to be the 'Superwoman'. Luckily for her this is not the case at all, the man does most of the work. In some ways the Superwoman position is quite like the Life Raft position.

The woman lies down on your bed on her belly, with her arms resting on the bed, stretched out in front of her. While her stomach should be on the bed, her waist will be at the edge with her legs hanging over the side. The man will then penetrate the woman while standing from behind and will start thrusting in and out.

Bulldog Sex Position

This position is similar in many ways to regular Doggy Style. However, this position puts the woman in an even more submissive position compare to the Doggy Style position. And makes you tighter for the man.

The woman gets down on all fours, on her hands and knees. Next she brings both of her legs together. The man then penetrates her from behind in a slight squatting position. He then places his feet outside of her legs and he can put his hands on the woman waist or her shoulders to steady himself.

Frog Leap Sex Position

In this position the woman squats, like a frog, in front of the man who kneels and penetrates from behind. The woman then arches her back to give easier access to the man, and the man should give a hand in supporting the weight of the woman as this position tends to lead to sore thighs for the woman in a short while.

Corner Doggy Style Sex Position

The sex position is a really great variation of the regular Doggy Style sex. While being performed on the corner of the bed or table, just like the similarly named Corner Cowgirl sex position, it has very little else in common with the position.

The woman starts off by standing upright on the floor with one of her legs positioned on either side of the corner of her bed or her table. The woman now leans over onto the bed or the table resting on either her elbows or her hands. Her man then enters her from behind, like he would during Bodyguard position or doggy Style position.

Bodyguard Sex Position

This position is a Spooning position with the fiery fire of the famous Doggy Style, the connectivity of a side by side position, and the erotic beauty that comes with the uniqueness of all standing positions.

The woman stands in front and is penetrated from behind by her man. This position is especially good in allowing the man access to touch and caress the woman's body. So make sure to keep those hands occupied!

The only difficulty with this position can be the alignment of the genitals which can be a real problem for some lovers.

It could be fixed by the following: standing on a foot stool, a stair, a couch cushion, or if the woman is up to it, maybe some high heels.

Bucking Bronco Sex Position

If you like being on top and having most of the control during sex then this sex position is great for you. The Bucking Bronco is very much like the Octopus position but is far easier and less exhausting to perform.

In this position, the man needs to lie down on his back. Then the woman needs to get on the top of him, facing him. When the man is inside the woman, she leans backwards and put her arms behind her to keep herself balanced. Then she puts her feet so that they are either side of the man's head. The wider she spreads her feet, the easier it will be to balance herself.

At this point, she will be able to bounce up and down on her man, just like a Bucking Bronco. She will find that it is quite easy to switch to the Bucking Bronco from the Reverse Cowgirl position.

Rear Admiral Sex Position

This position is great for those women that like to be dominated by their man. And in this position he is almost in complete control. The woman can perform this position while standing up or on her knees.

*while standing the couple faces in the same direction while both standing. The man now penetrates the woman from behind, either vaginally or anally. The woman now needs to bend over so that her stomach becomes parallel to the ground and she is facing the floor. The woman can spread her legs while the man keeps his own legs close together or vice-versa. Then the woman puts her arms parallel with her body. Her man then holds onto her hands or wrists and starts thrusting in and out.

In this position, your man can thrust in and out really hard and quite deep too if that's what you both enjoy.

*while on kneeling, the couples does everything as they would when they were standing, except that the couple will be on their knees. She spreads her knees wide and her man can keep his close together or vice/versa. The woman can also lean down a little and rest her head and shoulders on the bed if she likes.

That's the reason behind the name Rear Admiral. The man is in control of the 'ship' (the woman)

Stairway to Heaven

This position is also known as Step lively. This position is a variation on the Hot Seat with the woman sitting on top of her man while he sits on one of the stairs of a staircase! The Stairs offer very good seating possibilities and also a hand rail for lifting leverage and extra support.

Asian Cowgirl Sex Position

It is very similar to the regular cowgirl position. The woman stays on top; on the other hand the man lies down on his back. Though there are major differences that should be considered when performing it.

The woman has her knees either side of her man, resting on the bed in the regular cowgirl position. But when doing the Asian cowgirl with her man, the woman will be in a squatting position, which means that most of her weight is supported by her feet while she is squatting. She can use her hands to take some of her weight by putting them on either her man's chest or on either side of him on the bed. If she is not very strong or flexible, she will find the Asian cowgirl position to be exhaustive.

Fire Hydrant Sex Position

This position is a variant of the regular Doggy Style that some couples love while others are not so into it. To get into this position simply requires a little bit of flexibility.

The couple needs to get into the regular Doggy Style position. This means that the woman gets down on all fours, facing towards the floor. The man will then be on his knees behind her. He has to have his knees inside the woman's. The man is then going to have to start lifting one of his legs upwards and forwards and planting his foot on the floor to his woman's side. In so doing he will raise her leg on that side, so that her thigh will now be resting on top the man's thigh. This will make the woman look like a dog peeing on a fire hydrant.

Turtle Sex Position

This position is a type of Doggy Style sex position that requires a little bit of flexibility. It's a nice way to rev the excitement engines up when u start getting bored of the regular Doggy Style.

The woman rests with her knees on the floor. When in she's in this position, she lowers herself downwards so that her bum is sitting on top of the back of her ankles. Next she leans as far forward as she can possibly lean. She can grab hold of her legs in the front of her to help her lean further forward. Her man will be on his knees behind her thrusting into her. The man may find that he needs to adjust his height to make it easier for himself by either spreading his knees or bringing them together.

Bended Knee Sex Position

This position is a variation on the Dancer position; it is also a lot of fun if the couple is looking for something with face-to-face more intimate contact. The couples simply kneel facing each other. The woman simply raises one of her legs over the man's opposite thigh to give easier access while the man helps support her.

Book Ends Sex Position

This position comes really interesting. A lot of couples that wants to perform it may actually find it very difficult to penetrate comfortably. That's not to say that it's not a fun love making position though!

The couple would be on their knees facing each other on their bed. The man spreads out his knees so that he can lower himself while the woman will need to remain as tall as possible. When the man is then a little below her, he can now slide in his penis (the woman can be of helping, guiding in his penis). If it's comfortable, the man can then bring his legs together again and start to raise himself upwards. The woman can also lean backwards to make penetration deeper and more enjoyable for the man.

If the man is much taller than the woman, then she probably won't be able to perform actual penetrative sex in this sex position

Dublin Shuffle Sex Position

This position is one characterized with great fun and is great for lovers who value the intimacy of facing each other during sex along with the fun of both being upright while doing it. The reason it is called the Dublin Shuffle is because there is often a lot of shuffling when trying to find the exact right angle or 'spot'.

The man starts by standing on the floor, while the woman kneels on the bed. The couple will face each other. Before the couple goes any further, it is important to make certain that the base of his penis is at about the same height as her vagina. If not, the couple should put a few sturdy books under the bed to raise it, or the man should stand on something so that both the couples are at the right height. When the couple is both at a good height, the man can then penetrate her.

Shoe Shiner Sex Position

This position has a little bit in common with the Bended Knee Sex position as both the couple is facing each other while on just one knee.

The couple would face each other on their knees. They should be so close that they would be hugging each other. They are both going to raise their left knees so that their thighs are parallel to the bed and their lower legs are vertical with their left feet firmly on the bed. This will allow the man to penetrate her easily. If the man is a lot taller than the woman in this position, then the woman needs to put a pillow or a cushion under her knee to raise her high enough.

Teaspooning Sex Position

Teaspooning sex position is a variation of the regular Spooning position, and might actually be one of the most intimate sex positions of all time. It is also very easy to move from doggy-style position to this position.

The man gets to his knees on either the bed or the floor. He needs to open his knees fairly wide. The woman now gets on her knees also while facing in the same direction as her man in front of him.

The woman should have her knees together so that her man can come up close behind her and penetrate her. When he does, the man should wrap his arms around the woman. He can put them around her waist or on her breasts or under her arms to hold onto her shoulders.

After Dinner Sex Position

This position is somehow similar to the Back Seat Driver position. The name comes from the fact that you use a table and chair to perform it, making it perfect for right after dinner or after a meal.

The man needs to sit on a chair that is two feet from a table facing it, while his legs are open quite wide. The woman now needs to back herself up into her man with her legs quite close together in a standing position. Optionally, her man can then lift his legs up from the ground and place them on the table. Once he does this, the woman will be 'trapped' between his legs.

The Back Seat Driver Sex Position.

When having sex in this position, the man will sit on the edge of a sofa, a chair or even the bed with the man's legs spread wide and his feet on the floor. The woman now backs up onto your man's crotch and let him slowly thrust into her while bending her knees.

When the man is comfortably inside her, she will use her legs to bounce up and down on him. The couple will be facing in the same direction for this position.

Twister Sex Position

This position is a very exotic sex position, when you do it; it looks really out of this world. Well for the records just because a lovemaking position may be exotic, doesn't always mean that it is better. Also, just to be very clear, this position has nothing to do with the game called Twister.

The woman lies down on her side, probably her right side. The man will also be lying down on his right side, with his stomach facing the woman's stomach, but the woman will be laying head-to-toe with her man. This means that the head of the woman should be close to his feet. The couple needs to bend their left knees and raise them towards the ceiling. This will create a gap between his legs and the woman's leg.

The woman now leans forward and pushes her body through this gap so that her man's raised left leg is now above her waist, with the woman under it, but above his right leg. The woman will also be sandwiched between the man's legs with her left leg above his waist and right leg below. The man should now enter her and start thrusting.

If you think this looks complicated, you are very right, it is very complicated! It takes some practice before getting used to it.

Bouncing Spoon Sex Position

This position is a sort of pseudo-spooning position for couples. It is fairly easy to perform and a good option to liven up sex in the bedroom.

The man sits upright in bed with his back to the wall and his legs together and fairly straight (it doesn't have to be perfectly straight). The woman now needs to stand right over him with her back to him. Her feet should be on either side of his thighs. She then need to get down on her knees from this position and sit back onto the man's crotch and guide his penis inside her. She can now lean backwards so that her back is on her man's chest.

Lotus Sex Position

This position is a popular woman on top position, it is also called lotus blossom.

The man sits on the bed or floor in the lotus position, his legs crossed or extended. After he gets into position, the woman now straddles his lap and wraps her legs around his waist as he pushes into her, wrapping her arms around his torso for support. The woman can rock back and forth in this position for more pleasure. The position also allows intimate touches and kisses.

Mastery Sex Position

This is a great position that encourages intimacy, as it is very well face to face. That's good news for those that like a lot of kissing during sex. In this position the woman sits on man facing him. This position isn't great for generating vertical movement, so if you want to experience the full effect, it is important to try it on a stool or chair that lets the woman get a good footing.

See Saw Sex Position

This position is a really fun one, but couples get tired easily. There are really no similar positions to it, making it quite special. It also makes a good change from Doggy Style position or regular Missionary position.

The man sits on the bed. The woman then sits on his lap while facing her man. Next the woman should spread her legs out wide so that she is comfortable. She then needs to lean backwards and put her arms either on his shoulders or behind her. This position allows her to either move up and down on his penis or grind forwards and backwards on him all while facing her man.

Side Ride Sex Position

This position is basically a variation of the regular Asian Cowgirl position. It is very easy to perform and is good if the woman wants to be on top of her man during sex.

The man needs to lie down on his back like he would during the Cowgirl position. He would bend his knees slightly so that he can put his feet on the bed to give him some leverage for penetration. The woman now sits on her man's lap, allowing him to penetrate her. But instead of facing him or having her back to him, she is going to be sitting sideways on him. This means that she can sit on him with her feet on either the left side or the right side of him.

Side Saddle Sex Position

This position is superb for when the woman wants to be dominant and she just wants her man to relax and take it easy during sex. It's a great position to transfer to after blow-jobbing your man

The man lies down on his back on the bed. The man would have his butt at the edge of the bed with his legs hanging over it with his feet on the floor. He chooses how he positions his legs. Either together or spread out. The woman stands over her man with her back to him. She can sit down on top of him while spreading her legs if his legs are closed and together. But if he has his legs open then she would need to sit on top of him with her legs closed and together.

Final Furlong Sex Position

This position is a rear entry position that is physically very intimate. It is characterized by an ingenious use of an ottoman. It is similar to the teaspoon sex position.

The couples can replicate the sex position by hopping assuming the same stance a jockey would usually take in a race, by first mounting the 'saddle' (if the couple doesn't have an ottoman, a low couch arm can be used). The rear jockey which is the woman pulls the man in close and begins rocking his hips forward and back.

To create more movement and better penetration, the woman can raise herself off the ottoman slightly by simply putting more weight on her feet or leaning further forward. Be rest assured, there will be enough momentum gathered by the forward and backward motion to satisfy the woman's needs.

Carnal Crisscross

The woman starts by lying on her side with her arms above her head. The man on his side and his body perpendicular to the woman's, the woman slowly raises her top leg and let him inch his lower body between her legs. Once the couple is joined at the groin, the man should grab her shoulders while she anchors herself on the floor. The couple will need to hold on tight for this stellar trip!

END

Thank you for reading my book. If you enjoyed it, won't you please take a moment to look at my other titles?

Thanks!

Matt Elton